KIDNEY DISEASE RECIPES FOR NEWLY DIAGNOSED

1800 Days Tasty Recipes to Manage Kidney Health with Meal Plans Low in Sodium, Potassium, Phosphorus and Protein: 6-Weeks Quick & Easy Meal Plans.

EPIPHANY HUB PRINTS

KIDNEY DISEASE RECIPES FOR NEWLY DIAGNOSED

COPYRIGHT © [2023] BY [EPIPHANY HUB PRINTS]

TABLE OF CONTENT

INTRODUCTION

Living in a little village surrounded by bubbling brooks and undulating hills was a fascinating young cook named Mia. Mia has always had a love for cooking delectable meals that made people happy. But one beautiful day, she received an unexpected diagnosis of kidney disease for her close friend Alex, which turned her world upside down.

Mia set out on a culinary quest to find meals that were not only delicious but also specifically designed to fit the dietary requirements of individuals with renal illness, all in an effort to help Alex during this difficult journey. When Mia explored the world of kidney-friendly ingredients, she discovered a wealth of flavors that could turn any meal into a healthful celebration.

Mia's kitchen turned into a creative playground where she played around with vivid veggies, fresh herbs, and lean proteins to create foods that were not only good for the kidneys but also delicious. She found that cooking for kidney health may be a tasty and joyful undertaking when combined with a dash of creativity and a sprinkling of love.

Mia saw firsthand the healing effects of wholesome food on the body and the soul as she showed Alex her creations. Others who found themselves navigating the maze of kidney disease took inspiration from their culinary adventure. Mia came to the realization that a cookbook that would transform the kitchen into a haven for recently diagnosed individuals was desperately needed.

It led to the creation of "Kidney Disease Recipes for The Newly Diagnosed". In addition to delivering delicious recipes, this book tells the story of Mia and Alex's journey, giving hope and inspiration to anybody dealing with renal disease.

Every recipe serves as evidence for the idea that anybody can create a delicious and healthful haven in their kitchen with the correct ingredients and a dash of imagination. Let us embark on a gastronomic trip where each meal serves as a step towards well-being and each cuisine narrates a tale of resiliency and mouthwatering potential.

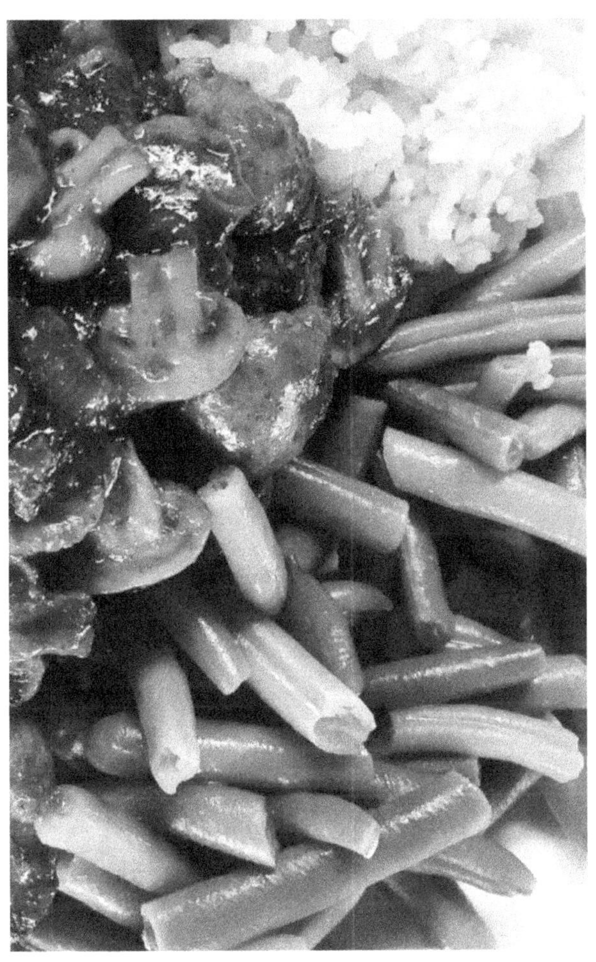

"EMBARK ON AN EXTRAORDINARY JOURNEY OF DISCOVERY AND ENLIGHTENMENT AS YOU DELVE INTO THE PAGES OF THIS CAPTIVATING BOOK, WHERE EACH CHAPTER UNFOLDS LIKE A HIDDEN TREASURE WAITING TO BE UNEARTHED, PROMISING TO IGNITE YOUR IMAGINATION, CHALLENGE YOUR PERCEPTIONS, AND LEAVE AN INDELIBLE MARK ON YOUR HEART AND MIND."

IN OUR BOOK SHELF WE'VE ALREADY CREATED

"THE ULTIMATE LOW CARB DIET RECIPES COOKBOOK FOR BEGINNERS"

HERE IS THE LINK …PLEASE CLICK!

"DIABETES BREAKFAST RECIPES MEAL PLAN FOR WOMEN"

HERE IS THE LINK….PLE ASE CLICK

"COMPLETE MEDITERRANEAN RECIPES COOKBOOK FOR SENIORS"

HERE IS THE LINK….PLEASE CLICK

CHAPTER 1: UNDERSTANDING KIDNEY DISEASE

Overview of the Role of Kidneys in the Body:

Maintaining the interior environment of the organism is mostly dependent on the kidneys. These are bean-shaped organs that are situated directly below the ribs on either side of the spine. The kidneys' primary purposes are as follows:

Blood Filtration: To create urine, the kidneys remove waste materials, extra ions, and fluids from the blood. This mechanism controls the body's fluid volume and aids in maintaining the appropriate balance of electrolytes, such as potassium and sodium.

Blood Pressure Regulation: The kidneys secrete a hormone known as renin, which affects the body's sodium and water balance to help control blood pressure.

Erythropoiesis Regulation: The kidneys secrete the hormone erythropoietin, which increases the bone marrow's ability to make red blood cells and contributes to the maintenance of a sufficient oxygen supply in the body.

Acid-Base Balance: **By eliminating hydrogen ions and reabsorbing bicarbonate ions, the kidneys assist in maintaining the body's acid-base equilibrium.**

Detoxification: **They rid the body of different medications and waste products, preventing the accumulation of dangerous substances.**

Functions of the Kidneys in Filtering and Eliminating Waste:

Nephrons are a sophisticated network of microscopic structures that carry out the waste filtering and removal process. About a million nephrons, each with its own filtering unit, make up each kidney. Among the crucial actions in trash removal are:

Filtration: **The glomerulus, a network of microscopic blood arteries inside the nephron, filters blood to separate waste materials from necessary components.**

Reabsorption: **The bloodstream reabsorbs necessary substances like glucose, water, and electrolytes.**

Secretion: **The urine actively draws in more waste materials from the blood.**

Excretion: **The last urine, which is made up of extra waste and water, is carried to the bladder where it is stored until the body gets rid of it.**

Kidney disease's common causes and risk factors are as follows:

Diabetes: Unchecked diabetes can eventually cause diabetic nephropathy, which damages the kidneys.

Hypertension: Prolonged high blood pressure can put stress on the kidneys, leading to nephron and blood vessel damage.

Genetics: Polycystic kidney disease is one of the genetic kidney illnesses.

Age: As people age, their risk of kidney disease rises.

Heart Disease: Problems with the heart may have an indirect effect on renal function.

Autoimmune Diseases: Kidney damage can result from autoimmune diseases such as lupus and others.

Infections: Certain acute infections as well as chronic kidney infections might aggravate renal illness.

Kidney Disease Recipes for the Newly Diagnosed:

Dietary changes might be required if renal disease is just discovered. Controlling the consumption of protein, salt, potassium, and phosphorus is essential. The following general rules apply:

Low-Protein Recipes: Put an emphasis on high-quality, low-protein foods like eggs, fish, and chicken. Limit your red meat. Look into recipes that use grains and legumes.

Low-Sodium Recipes: Use herbs and spices to provide flavor instead of salt. Whole grains, lean meats, and fresh produce are all healthy options.

Low-Potassium Recipes: Select foods such as apples, berries, and cauliflower that are lower in potassium. To lower the potassium level of high-potassium foods, cook or soak them.

Management of Phosphorus: Restrict dairy and high-phosphorus processed foods. Select recipes that call for low-phosphorus substitutes.

Fluid Control: Control your fluid intake by choosing recipes that call for little to no additional fluids. Be careful—soups and stews might increase your fluid intake.

The Importance of Nutrition in Kidney Care

Recognizing the vital link between nutrition and kidney health

Maintaining general health, particularly in the setting of renal illness, requires an understanding of the critical relationship between diet and kidney health. The kidneys are essential for controlling electrolyte balance, removing waste and extra fluid from the blood, and sustaining general metabolic processes. As a result, food decisions directly affect kidney function; individuals with kidney illness must comprehend this relationship.

1. Understanding the Impact of Dietary Choices:

Consumption of Salt: Consuming too much salt can raise blood pressure, which further strains the kidneys. Salt restriction is frequently necessary for those with kidney illness in order to control blood pressure and lower their chance of fluid retention.

Consumption of Protein: Although protein is necessary, consuming too much of it might damage the kidneys. For those with renal illness, managing the kind and quantity of protein is essential. Plant-based, high-quality proteins are frequently advised.

2. Exploring Nutrients Essential for Supporting Kidney Function:

Fluid Balance: Healthy kidney function depends on drinking enough water. In the form of urine, water aids the kidneys in eliminating waste from the circulation. However, depending on their particular condition, people with kidney disease may need to control how much fluid they consume.

Electrolytes: It's critical to preserve the equilibrium of electrolytes, such as potassium and phosphorus. Dietary recommendations frequently include monitoring and regulating the intake of foods rich in these minerals because imbalances can result in difficulties.

Dietary Restrictions and Guidelines

Overview of dietary restrictions for individuals with kidney disease

Kidney disease patients frequently require special food regimens to help control their illness and stop future kidney damage. This is a summary of the food rules that apply to people with renal disease. It includes recommendations for controlling the amount of protein, sodium, and potassium consumed as well as the significance of keeping an eye on the amounts of fluid and phosphorus in the diet. For those who are freshly diagnosed, I will also offer some recipes that are kidney-friendly.

Protein Intake:

Recommendation: Eat less protein because too much protein can strain the kidneys.

Reasoning: Restricting protein helps lessen the burden on the kidneys since protein metabolism generates waste that the kidneys must filter.

Sodium (Salt) Intake:

Recommendation: Cut back on sodium to control blood pressure and maintain fluid equilibrium.

Reasoning: Elevated blood pressure and fluid retention are two consequences of high salt levels that can harm kidney function.

Potassium Intake:

Recommendation: Control potassium intake since excessive consumption may be detrimental to the heart.

Reasoning: Potassium levels may be difficult for impaired kidneys to maintain equilibrium, which raises the risk of cardiac issues.

Phosphorus Monitoring:

Recommendation: Monitor phosphorus consumption since kidney impairment may make it difficult for the body to eliminate too much of it.

Reasoning: In patients with renal impairment, elevated phosphorus levels may be a factor in cardiac and bone problems.

Fluid Control:

Recommendation: Keep an eye on your fluid intake to avoid swelling and fluid retention.

The objective is: Damaged kidneys may have trouble maintaining the proper balance of fluids, which can result in edema and elevated blood pressure.

Importance of Monitoring Phosphorus and Fluid Levels:

Phosphorus:

Significance: High phosphorus levels may cause cardiac problems, hardening of blood vessels, and problems with bones.

Watching: Select foods with less phosphorus and think about taking phosphorus binders as directed by a medical practitioner.

Fluid Levels:

Relevance: Hypertension, edema, and issues with the heart and lungs can result from fluid retention.

Monitoring: Adhere to certain fluid limitations, taking into consideration the amount of fluid in meals, and seek the guidance of healthcare professionals.

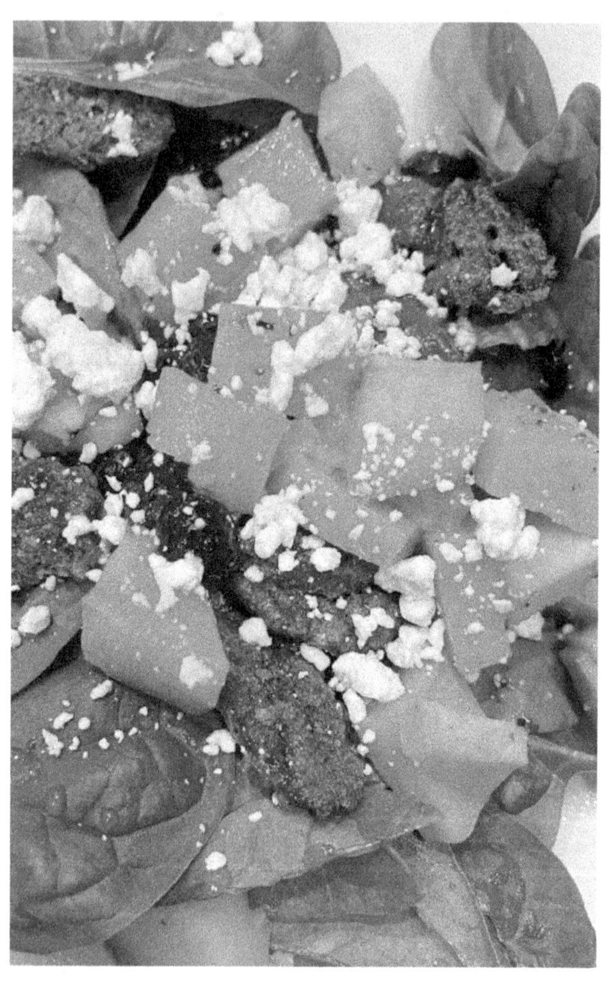

CHAPTER 2:
BREAKFASTS FOR KIDNEY HEALTH

Low-Phosphorus Smoothie Bowl:

Ingredients:

Berries: Not only are blueberries, strawberries, and raspberries tasty, but they are also low in phosphorus.

Banana: A naturally sweet fruit that is high in potassium.

Greek yogurt (low-phosphorus): To maintain the smoothie bowl kidney-friendly, go for a yogurt that has less phosphorus.

Unsweetened almond milk: A dairy substitute with little phosphorus.

Chia seeds: They don't raise phosphorus levels and can provide texture and nutritional benefits.

Explanation:

Phosphorus control is essential for kidney health. High phosphorus levels can contribute to bone and heart issues in individuals with kidney disease. This smoothie bowl is a tasty and low-phosphorus option, incorporating nutrient-rich fruits and low-phosphorus dairy alternatives.

Egg White Omelette with Vegetables:

Ingredients:

Egg whites: A source of protein devoid of phosphorus, as opposed to egg yolks.

Low-potassium vegetables: Such as bell peppers, spinach, tomatoes, and onions contribute taste and nutrition.

Herbs and spices: To enhance taste without adding extra sodium, use herbs like dill or parsley.

Explanation

Egg yolks contain phosphorus, while egg whites offer a superior source of protein. Because spinach and bell peppers are low in potassium, people with kidney problems can safely eat this omelette. You may improve the flavor without consuming more sodium by adding herbs and spices.

Quinoa Breakfast Porridge:

Ingredients:

Quinoa: A grain high in protein and low in phosphorus when compared to some other grains.

Unsweetened almond milk: A dairy substitute with little phosphorus content.

Nutmeg and cinnamon: These spices enhance flavor without raising blood pressure.

Fresh fruit, such as berries or apples: Can offer extra nutrients and a naturally pleasant taste.

Explanation

Because quinoa has less phosphorus than typical grains, it's a good substitute. You may make a tasty and nutritious breakfast by cooking it as a porridge with almond milk and adding spices for taste. Fresh fruit is added to provide extra vitamins and a natural sweetness.

CHAPTER 3:
SATISFYING LUNCH OPTIONS

Of course! It's crucial to consider the nutritional content while developing lunch meals for people with renal illness, particularly with regard to protein, phosphorus, salt, and potassium. The following are adapted recipes for the dishes listed:

Grilled Lemon Herb Chicken Salad:

Ingredients:

Four skinless and boneless chicken breasts

Two tsp of olive oil

One lemon, juiced

Two minced garlic cloves

One tsp of dehydrated oregano

One tsp of dehydrated basil

Add pepper and salt to taste.

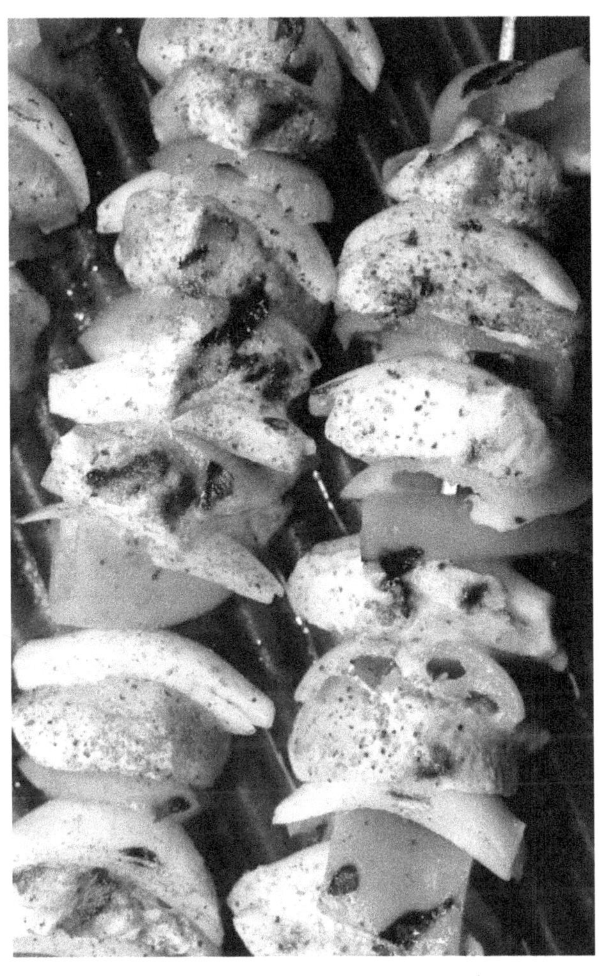

Mixed salad greens, such as Romaine, red leaf lettuce, or iceberg lettuce (low-potassium variants)

Bell peppers, cucumber slices, and cherry tomatoes (choose low-potassium varieties)

Balsamic vinaigrette (low-sodium)

Instructions:

Make a marinade in a bowl by combining olive oil, lemon juice, minced garlic, dried oregano, dried basil, salt, and pepper.

For a minimum of half an hour, marinate the chicken breasts in this mixture.

Cook the chicken completely on the grill.

Slicing the grilled chicken, it is served with low-potassium veggies on a bed of mixed salad greens.

Drizzle with a balsamic vinaigrette that is low in salt.

Vegetarian Chickpea and Spinach Stew:

Ingredients:

Two cans of rinsed and drained low-sodium chickpeas

One tsp of olive oil

Chop one onion.

Two minced garlic cloves

One tsp cumin

One teaspoon of cilantro

One tsp of paprika

Four cups of fresh spinach, or greens low in potassium

4 cups of vegetable broth with minimal sodium

Add pepper and salt to taste.

Instruction

Add the garlic and onions to a large pot and sauté in olive oil until tender.

Stir in paprika, coriander, cumin, and chickpeas. Mix thoroughly.

After adding the vegetable broth, boil the mixture.

Add the spinach when it starts to wilt.

Season with salt and pepper, to taste.

Salmon and Asparagus Quinoa Bowl:

Ingredients:

Four fillets of salmon

Two tsp of olive oil

One lemon, juiced

Two tsp Dijon mustard

Two cups prepared quinoa

1 clipped bunch of asparagus

Zest of lemon for garnish

Add pepper and salt to taste.

Instruction

Set oven temperature to 400°F, or 200°C.

Whisk together lemon juice, Dijon mustard, and olive oil in a small bowl.

After putting the salmon fillets on a baking sheet, sprinkle them with salt and pepper and drizzle them with the lemon-mustard sauce.

Place the asparagus next to the fish.

Bake until the fish is cooked through and the asparagus is soft.

Serve with lemon zest as a garnish over quinoa.

These recipes emphasize the use of low-potassium, fresh foods without sacrificing flavor for those with renal illness. For those who have renal problems, speaking with a medical expert or a trained dietitian is crucial in order to customize their diet to meet their individual requirements.

CHAPTER 4:

FLAVORFUL DINNERS WITHOUT COMPROMISE

Baked Cod with Lemon-Dill Sauce:

Ingredients:

Four fillets of cod

Two tsp of olive oil

Add pepper and salt to taste.

Two squeezed lemons

One tablespoon of freshly chopped dill

1 tsp powdered garlic

Kidney-compatible Adjustments:

To lower the sodium content, choose fresh fish and clean it.

For taste, use herbs and spices rather than too much salt.

To manage potassium levels, cut back on lemon juice.

Instructions:

Turn the oven on to 375°F, or 190°C.

Cod fillets should be put on a baking pan.

After drizzling the fillets with olive oil, season them with lemon juice, salt, pepper, and garlic powder.

Bake the fish for 15 to 20 minutes, or until it flake easily.

Before serving, scatter some fresh dill over the top.

Turkey and Vegetable Stir-Fry:

Ingredients:

Turkey ground, 1 pound, lean

Two cups florets of broccoli

One bell pepper, cut thinly

One sliced zucchini

Two tsp of soy sauce (low sodium)

1 tsp finely chopped ginger

two minced garlic cloves

One tsp of sesame oil

Kidney-compatible Adjustments:

To cut down on saturated fat, choose lean turkey.

To reduce your intake of sodium, use low-sodium soy sauce.

Cut back on garlic and ginger to control potassium levels.

Instructions:

Brown the ground turkey over medium heat in a large skillet.

To the skillet, add the bell pepper, zucchini, and broccoli.

Stir in the soy sauce, ginger, and garlic.

Sauté the vegetables until they are crisp-tender.

Before serving, drizzle the stir-fry with sesame oil.

Pasta with Broccoli and Cauliflower:

Ingredients:

Two cups florets of cauliflower

Two cups florets of broccoli

8 ounces of low-phosphorus or whole-grain pasta

One cup of nonfat milk

Grated Parmesan cheese, one cup

Two minced garlic cloves

Add pepper and salt to taste.

Kidney-friendly Adjustments:

Select pasta with reduced phosphorus content.

To cut down on saturated fat, choose low-fat milk.

Use a modest quantity of Parmesan to reduce your sodium intake.

Instructions:

Cook the pasta according to the package's instructions.

Broccoli and cauliflower should be steamed till soft.

Steamed veggies, milk, Parmesan, garlic, salt, and pepper should all be combined in a blender. Mix until homogeneous.

Mix the Alfredo sauce with the cooked pasta.

Serve after adding a little extra Parmesan cheese on top.

Don't forget to speak with a medical expert or a renal dietician to make sure these recipes fit the particular dietary needs of the kidney disease sufferer.

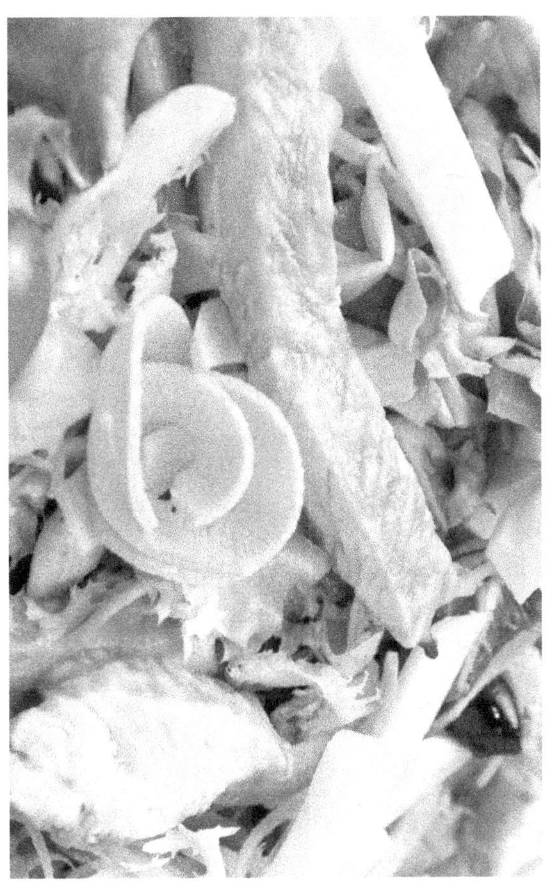

CHAPTER 5:
SNACKING SMARTLY FOR KIDNEY HEALTH

Roasted Red Pepper Hummus with Fresh Veggies:

Ingredients:

One can (15 ounces) of rinsed and drained chickpeas

Half a cup tahini

1/4 cup juice from lemons

Two minced garlic cloves

Half a teaspoon of cumin powder

One-fourth cup of extra virgin olive oil

Add pepper and salt to taste.

One cup of raw vegetables, such as cherry tomatoes, cucumber slices, and carrot sticks

Kidney Health Factors to Consider:

Plant-based protein, which is generally advised for kidney health, is present in chickpeas.

Tahini offers good fats, but because it contains phosphorus, you must watch your portion sizes.

Fresh vegetables don't raise potassium or phosphorus levels; instead, they add vitamins and minerals.

Baked Sweet Potato Chips:

Ingredients:

Two medium sweet potatoes, sliced very thinly

One or two teaspoons olive oil

One-half tsp paprika

One-half tsp of garlic powder

Add salt to taste.

Kidney Health Factors to Consider:

Sweet potatoes are less potassium-rich than normal potatoes, making them kinder to the kidneys.

Baking rather than frying saves extra oil and keeps everything kidney-friendly.

Garlic powder and paprika are examples of spices that enhance flavor without endangering kidney health.

Greek Yogurt Parfait with Berries:

Ingredients:

One cup Greek yogurt (low-fat)

Half a cup of mixed berries, including raspberries, strawberries, and blueberries

One spoonful of agave syrup or honey

One-fourth cup of low-phosphorus granola

Kidney Health Factors to Consider:

Greek yogurt can be incorporated into a diet that is kidney-friendly and is a fantastic source of high-quality protein.

Berries are abundant in antioxidants and low in potassium.

You can choose a granola that has less phosphorus in it or not at all.

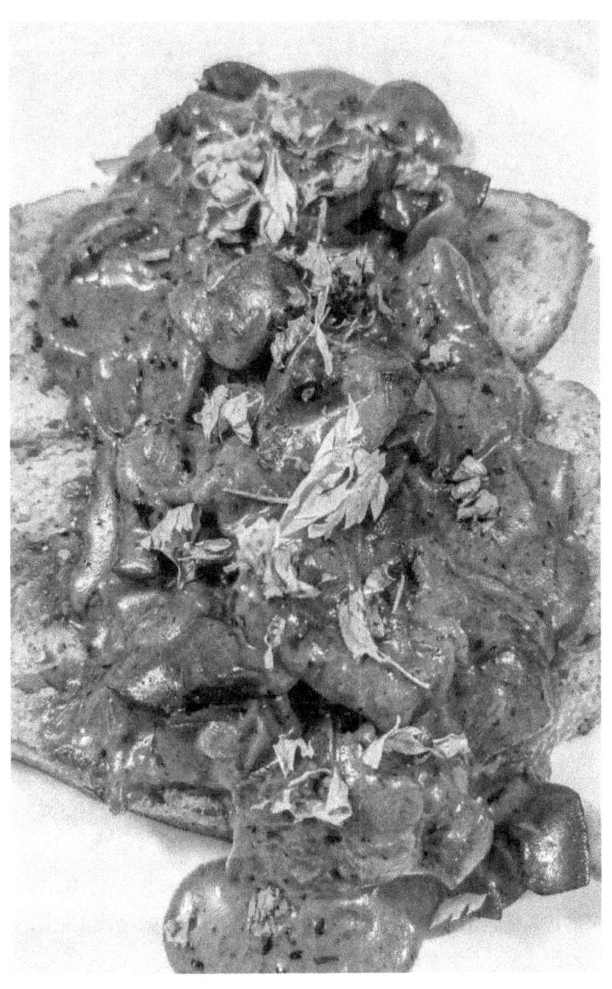

CHAPTER 6:

KIDNEY-FRIENDLY DESSERTS

Desserts that are suitable for people with kidney illness are made to meet their dietary preferences and medical requirements. The main goal of these sweets is to restrict specific nutrients—such as potassium, sodium, and phosphorus—which are frequently limited in a diet that is kidney-friendly. This is a detailed rundown of all the desserts that were mentioned:

Berry and Chia Seed Pudding:

Ingredients:

Berries: Generally speaking, berries—strawberries, raspberries, and blueberries—have less potassium than other fruits.

Chia seeds: Rich in protein, fiber, and omega-3 fatty acids without adding a lot of potassium.

Lower in phosphorus than cow's milk is almond or rice milk.

Sweetener: In moderation, use a kidney-friendly sweetener, like a tiny bit of honey or a sugar replacement.

Instruction

Chia seeds should be combined with rice or almond milk and left to soak overnight.

Arrange fresh berries on top of the chia pudding.

After adding sugar to taste, chill the mixture until it takes on the consistency of pudding.

Taking into account

To limit nutrient intake, pay attention to portion sizes.

Adapt sweetness to your own taste.

Banana-Oat Cookies:

Ingredients:

Oats rolled: A wholesome fiber source.

For natural sweetness in mashed bananas, use ripe bananas.

Egg whites or egg substitute: Used in place of whole eggs to lower the phosphorus level.

Cinnamon: Flavors food without contributing much in the way of nutrients.

Instruction

Combine cinnamon, rolled oats, egg substitute, and mashed bananas.

Once they are browned, drop spoonfuls onto a baking sheet and bake.

Taking into account

To reduce your consumption of potassium, eat fewer cookies.

To lower phosphorus, use egg whites or egg alternatives.

Mango and Mint Sorbet:

Ingredients:

Mangoes that are ripe: Full of vitamins and flavor.

Lemon juice: Adds sourness without greatly raising potassium levels.

Fresh mint: Enhances flavor without raising any nutritional issues.

Instruction

Smoothly blend ripe mangos with lemon juice.

Blend again after adding fresh mint.

To achieve a sorbet texture, freeze the mixture in a shallow pan or an ice cream machine, stirring from time to time.

Taking into account

Consume in moderation to control your intake of potassium.

For naturally sweet mangoes, choose ripe ones.

CHAPTER 7:

MANAGING FLUID INTAKE WITH REFRESHING DRINKS

Controlling fluid consumption is essential for those with renal disease. Maintaining an appropriate level of hydration supports renal function and guards against problems brought on by fluid imbalance.

Here, we'll look at three cool beverages that can be incorporated into a kidney-friendly diet for people who have recently been diagnosed with kidney disease: watermelon lime slush, hibiscus iced tea, and cucumber and mint infused water.

Cucumber and Mint Infused Water:

Ingredients:

Cut up cucumbers

Water

Fresh mint leaves

Benefits:

Because they are low in potassium, cucumbers are a good choice for people who have kidney problems.

Mint gives a flavor that is both refreshing and low in calories and potentially dangerous ingredients.

Instruction

Cucumbers should be sliced and added to a pitcher.

Assemble new mint leaves.

Pour water into the pitcher and refrigerate for a few hours to allow the flavor to infuse.

Tips for Success:

Change the amounts of cucumber and mint to adjust the taste strength.

This flavor-infused water encourages proper hydration by offering a delightful substitute for regular water.

Tea with Hibiscus Ice:

Ingredients:

Dried hibiscus petals or hibiscus tea bags

Lemon slices (optional) with water

Benefits:

There may be advantages to drinking hibiscus tea for kidney health, such as reduced blood pressure.

It's a caffeine-free choice that's appropriate for people with kidney problems.

Instruction

Steep the tea bags or petals in boiling water to make hibiscus tea.

Refrigerate after letting it cool.

If preferred, serve with lemon slices and over ice.

Advice:

Keep an eye on how much tea you drink because too much tea can raise your potassium levels.

Watermelon Lime Slush:

Ingredients:

Seedless watermelon pieces, lime juice, and ice cubes.

Benefits:

A fruit with a high water content that is hydrating is watermelon.

Lime gives food a zesty taste without having a big effect on renal health.

Instruction

Puree the chunks of watermelon till smooth.

As desired, add lime juice.

Blend once more with ice cubes to achieve a slushy texture.

Tips for Success:

To save time and trouble picking out the seeds, go for seedless watermelon.

To suit your tastes, add or subtract lime juice.

It's important to take into account any dietary restrictions when including these drinks in a kidney-friendly diet. To customize these recipes to meet particular needs, speak with a licensed dietitian or healthcare practitioner. Furthermore, it is essential for people with renal disease to manage their fluid intake and adhere to established limits in order to preserve their general health and wellbeing.

CHAPTER 8:

TIPS FOR DINING OUT AND SPECIAL OCCASIONS

Obviously! It's critical to manage kidney health, particularly for people who have just received a kidney disease diagnosis. The following are some pointers and recommendations for socializing, dining out, navigating restaurant menus, cooking for special events, and dining out without endangering kidney health:

Select Restaurants That Are Kidney-Friendly:

Seek out eateries that have kidney-friendly and healthful menu items. These days, a lot of places provide nutritional information, which can assist you in making wise decisions.

Make a Plan:

Before you go, check out the restaurant's online menu. This helps you recognize kidney-friendly options so you may choose more wisely.

Explain Dietary Limitations:

Tell the cook or waiter about your renal condition and the restrictions on your diet. They frequently agree to fulfill unique demands.

Portion sizes to watch:

Pay attention to portion sizes because excessive consumption of minerals like potassium and phosphorus, which should be restricted in kidney disease, might result from large servings.

Limiting Foods Rich in Potassium and Phosphorus:

Select dishes from the menu that are lower in phosphorus and potassium. This can entail staying away from particular dressings, sauces, and processed meals.

Navigating Restaurant Menus:

Opt for Grilled or Baked Options:

Instead of frying proteins, opt for grilling or baking them because frying can result in an accumulation of undesirable fats and salt.

Select Side Dishes Carefully:

Steer clear of high-potassium sauces and garnishes when ordering pasta, rice, or steamed veggies.

Take Care When Adding Condiments:

Keep an eye out for condiments that are heavy in sodium because consuming too much salt can be harmful to the kidneys.

Ask for Adjustments:

Never be afraid to request adjustments to accommodate your dietary requirements. The majority of eateries are welcoming.

Cooking for Special Occasions:

Experiment with Kidney-Friendly Recipes:

Look at recipes with little salt, potassium, and phosphorus content. There are many of delectable options that can still provide enjoyment to special events.

Use Fresh Ingredients:

Include fresh produce in your meals as it is typically lower in salt and other unhealthy substances.

Eat Fewer Processed Foods:

Reduce your intake of processed foods because they frequently have additives that could not be good for your kidneys.

Making Friends without Endangering Your Kidney Health:

Bring Your Own Food, or BYOF,:

Consider bringing a food that is kidney-friendly to offer if you are attending an event. This guarantees that you will always have a safe choice.

Stay Hydrated:

It's important to be well hydrated since it supports healthy kidneys. If you have fluid limits, though, pay attention to how much fluid you consume.

Educate Your Friends and Family:

Inform your loved ones about your dietary needs so they can be accommodating when it comes to organizing get-togethers or meals.

CONCLUSION

Kidney disease might feel like a plot twist in the magical realm of wellness, where our bodies are the heroes of our journeys. Nevertheless, do not be alarmed, brave readers; all heroes require the proper fuel to start their path to recovery. As we come to the end of our investigation into kidney-friendly meals for recently diagnosed individuals, let's envision a gastronomic journey full of tastes that revitalize and mend.

Imagine a magical kitchen where ingredients work in unison to create recipes that nourish the powerful kidneys in addition to pleasing the taste buds. Every recipe, from colorful salads to flavorful stews, is a concoction that has been meticulously mixed to support our brave organs as they heal.

Therefore, my dear friends, keep in mind that the quest for wellness is a never-ending story as you turn the final page of this culinary adventure. With these kidney-friendly recipes at your disposal, may your kitchen turn into a haven of healing and may your taste buds celebrate their delectable triumph over hardship. Cheers to a bright, tasty, and well-being-filled future!